HISTAMINE INTOLERANCE

Your Comprehensive Guide To Relief with Symptoms, Diagnosis, Treatment Options, Recovery Strategies, and Meal Plan Inspirations

Dr Andy Brighton

Table of Contents

WHAT TO EXPECT

Dear Readers,

Welcome to HISTAMINE INTOLERANCE: Your Comprehensive Guide To Relief with Symptoms, Diagnosis, Treatment Options, Recovery Strategies, and Meal Plan Inspirations." We are thrilled to embark on this journey with you as we explore the intricate world of histamine intolerance and equip you with the knowledge and tools necessary to navigate this condition effectively.

In this book, we delve deep into the complexities of histamine intolerance, shedding light on its causes, symptoms, diagnosis, treatment options, and practical strategies for living well despite its challenges. Whether you're newly diagnosed or have been grappling with histamine intolerance for years, this book is designed to be your trusted companion, offering insights, guidance, and support every step of the way.

Here's what you can expect to find within the pages of this comprehensive guide:

1. Understanding Histamine Intolerance: We kick off our exploration by delving into the fundamentals of histamine intolerance, including its definition, underlying mechanisms, and who is most affected by this condition. By laying a solid foundation of understanding, you'll be better equipped to navigate the complexities that lie ahead.

2. Symptoms and Diagnosis: We take a detailed look at the wide array of symptoms associated with histamine intolerance, from the commonly recognized to the lesser-known manifestations. You'll learn how to recognize these symptoms in yourself or others and understand the process of diagnosis, including medical

history assessment, symptom tracking, and diagnostic tests.

3. Causes and Triggers: Unravelling the mysteries of histamine intolerance wouldn't be complete without exploring its root causes and triggers. From enzyme deficiencies to dietary factors and environmental influences, we examine the multifaceted factors that contribute to histamine intolerance and how they interact to produce symptoms.

4. Treatment and Management: Armed with knowledge about the causes and triggers of histamine intolerance, we dive into the various treatment options and management strategies available. From dietary modifications and supplementation to medications and alternative therapies, you'll discover practical approaches to alleviate symptoms and improve your quality of life.

5. Living Well with Histamine Intolerance: Beyond managing symptoms, we explore the practicalities of living with histamine intolerance day-to-day. From navigating social situations to travelling and dining out, you'll find valuable tips and strategies for maintaining a fulfilling life while managing this condition.

6. Recovery and Long-Term Management: We guide you through the journey of recovery from histamine intolerance, outlining a phased approach to healing, monitoring progress, and making long-term dietary adjustments. You'll learn how to reintroduce foods safely and stay informed to ensure sustained well-being.

7. Practical Resources: To support you on your journey, we provide a wealth of practical resources, including meal plans, recipes, a glossary of terms, frequently asked questions, comprehensive food lists, and a sample food diary template. These

resources are designed to empower you to make informed choices and take control of your health.

As you embark on this enlightening and empowering journey through the pages of "Navigating Histamine Intolerance: A Comprehensive Guide," we encourage you to approach it with an open mind and a willingness to embrace new insights and strategies. Remember, you are not alone in your journey, and together, we can navigate histamine intolerance with confidence and resilience.

Wishing you health, happiness, and empowerment on your path ahead.

Sincerely,

Dr Andy Brighton

TRIGGER, TAME, TRIUMPH (An Overview)

When I first heard the term "histamine intolerance," I admit, my initial reaction was confusion. Histamine? Isn't that something to do with allergies? Like the stuff in antihistamines that we take for hay fever? If you're feeling the same way, let me reassure you—you're not alone. The concept of histamine intolerance is relatively new and often misunderstood, even among health professionals. But don't worry; by the time you finish this book, you'll be well-versed in everything histamine-related. And who knows? You might even become the go-to person in your circle for all things histamine!

So, what exactly is histamine intolerance? Think of histamine as a kind of bouncer at the doors of your body's party. It's a naturally occurring compound that plays a key role in your immune system, your gut, and your central nervous system. When everything's working as it should, histamine helps regulate physiological function and works as a neurotransmitter. It's involved in immune responses, regulating stomach acid, and communicating messages from your body to your brain. Essentially, histamine is like the life of the party—keeping things lively and in order.

But what happens when the bouncer starts to misbehave? When histamine levels get too high or when your body can't break it down properly, that's when problems start. Picture this: the party is going great, but suddenly, more and more people show up. The bouncer is overwhelmed, and chaos ensues. This is essentially what happens in your body when you have histamine intolerance. The excess histamine causes a range of symptoms that can make you feel miserable.

Histamine intolerance isn't exactly a disease or an allergy. It's more of a condition where your body accumulates too much histamine, either because it produces too much or can't break it down efficiently. Normally, our bodies produce enzymes, like diamine oxidase (DAO) and histamine-N-methyltransferase (HNMT), to metabolize and get rid of excess histamine. But for various reasons, sometimes our systems can't keep up.

You might be wondering, what causes this imbalance? Well, there's no one-size-fits-all answer. It could be due to genetic factors, where you naturally have lower levels of the enzymes needed to break down histamine. It could be linked to gut health issues, where conditions like leaky gut or dysbiosis (an imbalance in gut bacteria) affect your ability to manage histamine levels. Even certain medications and lifestyle factors can play a role.

Living with histamine intolerance can feel like trying to navigate a minefield. Symptoms can vary widely from person to person, making it a bit of a detective game to figure out what's going on. Common symptoms include headaches, migraines, digestive issues like bloating and diarrhea, skin problems such as hives and eczema, and respiratory issues like nasal congestion or asthma. Some people even experience anxiety, dizziness, or an irregular heartbeat. It's like your body is sending out distress signals, but they're all mixed up.

My journey into understanding histamine intolerance started with a series of seemingly unrelated health issues. I had always prided myself on being relatively healthy, but suddenly, I found myself battling frequent headaches, unexplained rashes, and bouts of stomach discomfort. At first, I dismissed these as minor annoyances, chalking them up to stress or something I ate. But as time went on, the symptoms became more persistent and harder to ignore. I began to feel like a shadow of my former self, constantly fatigued and on edge.

Determined to get to the bottom of it, I embarked on what felt like an epic quest for answers. I visited multiple doctors, underwent various tests, and tried different treatments, but nothing seemed to add up. It was only after stumbling upon an article about histamine intolerance that the pieces of the puzzle started to fit together. Here was something that explained not just one or two of my symptoms, but all of them. It was a lightbulb moment.

Learning about histamine intolerance was like discovering a hidden chapter of my health story. It wasn't an easy journey, but it was empowering. I started to educate myself about the condition, diving into medical journals, books, and online forums. I experimented with my diet, carefully noting which foods seemed to trigger symptoms and which ones didn't. I began to understand the importance of gut health and the role it played in managing histamine levels. Slowly but surely, I started to feel better.

One of the most surprising things I learned was how common histamine intolerance might be, yet how often it goes undiagnosed. Many people, just like I did, suffer from a range of vague and seemingly unrelated symptoms for years without realizing that histamine could be the culprit. That's why I decided to write this book. I wanted to create a comprehensive, accessible guide to help others understand histamine intolerance, recognize its symptoms, and find ways to manage it effectively.

Imagine waking up one day without the nagging headache, the relentless itch, or the constant stomach upset. Imagine feeling more like yourself again, with more energy and less anxiety. That's the goal. I want to take you by the hand and lead you through the maze of histamine intolerance. Together, we'll explore the science behind it, discuss the various symptoms and their triggers, and look at practical ways to manage and reduce your histamine levels.

This book isn't just about information—it's about transformation. It's about empowering you with knowledge and giving you the tools to take control of your health. We'll delve into the nitty-gritty of dietary changes, explore the benefits of different supplements, and even look at lifestyle adjustments that can make a big difference. I'll share meal plans and recipes to help you navigate the world of low-histamine eating without feeling deprived. And because every journey is unique, I'll include personal stories and testimonials from others who have walked this path, so you know you're not alone.

So, whether you're newly diagnosed, suspect you might have histamine intolerance, or are simply curious about the condition, this book is for you. It's a guide, a companion, and a source of support as you work towards better health. My hope is that, by the end of our time together, you'll not only have a clearer understanding of histamine intolerance but also a practical plan to manage it and reclaim your life.

Let's embark on this journey together. Here's to understanding, healing, and thriving. Welcome to the world of histamine intolerance. Let's get started.

CHAPTER 1: Understanding Histamine Intolerance

What is Histamine Intolerance?

Imagine you're enjoying a lovely dinner with friends, savoring a glass of red wine and a plate of aged cheese. Suddenly, you feel a wave of discomfort: a headache sets in, your skin flushes, and your stomach churns. You might brush it off as an allergy or just bad luck, but these could be signs of histamine intolerance.

Histamine intolerance is a condition that occurs when there's an imbalance between the histamine you ingest or produce and your body's ability to break it down. Unlike food allergies, which trigger an immune response, histamine intolerance results from an accumulation of histamine, leading to various symptoms. Essentially, it's your body telling you it's overwhelmed by this naturally occurring chemical.

The Role of Histamine in the Body

Histamine is a biogenic amine, a type of chemical that plays multiple roles in your body. It's a crucial player in your immune response, acting as a messenger to help your body deal with allergens. When you come into contact with something you're allergic to, histamine is released from mast cells, leading to familiar allergic symptoms like itching, sneezing, and swelling.

But histamine's job doesn't end there. It's also involved in regulating stomach acid production, helping you digest food, and acting as a neurotransmitter, communicating important signals between your brain and your body. In small, controlled amounts, histamine is your ally, aiding in critical bodily functions.

Causes and Mechanisms

The primary cause of histamine intolerance is a deficiency or dysfunction of the enzymes that break down histamine—diamine oxidase (DAO) and histamine-N-methyltransferase (HNMT). DAO primarily works in your gut, breaking down histamine from the food you eat, while HNMT functions mainly in your tissues, managing the histamine produced within your body.

Several factors can impede these enzymes' ability to do their job. Genetic predispositions can play a part, meaning you might be born with lower levels of these enzymes. Certain medications, such as antibiotics, antidepressants, and antihypertensives, can inhibit DAO activity. Additionally, gastrointestinal disorders like leaky gut, Crohn's disease, and irritable bowel syndrome can reduce enzyme production or release, further complicating histamine breakdown.

Understanding Histamine Intolerance: A Growing Concern

Histamine intolerance is gaining recognition as more people report symptoms that don't fit into neat diagnostic categories. This condition is often overlooked or misdiagnosed because its symptoms mimic those of other common ailments. However, with increased awareness and research, we're beginning to understand its prevalence and impact better.

Histamine intolerance can manifest in various ways, making it a chameleon of sorts in the medical world. Symptoms can range from headaches, migraines, and digestive issues to skin reactions like hives and eczema, respiratory problems such as asthma and nasal congestion, and even neurological symptoms like anxiety and dizziness. Because these symptoms are so diverse and can overlap with other conditions, many people go through a lengthy and frustrating process before getting a proper diagnosis.

Who is Affected by Histamine Intolerance?

Histamine intolerance doesn't discriminate—it can affect anyone, regardless of age, gender, or ethnicity. However, certain groups may be more susceptible. Women, for example, often report symptoms more frequently than men, potentially due to hormonal influences on histamine levels. Estrogen, for instance, can increase histamine release and reduce DAO activity, which might explain why some women experience heightened symptoms during their menstrual cycles or pregnancy.

Individuals with pre-existing gastrointestinal conditions are also at higher risk. Since DAO is produced in the gut, any disorder that affects gut health can impact DAO levels and, consequently, histamine breakdown. This includes conditions like irritable bowel syndrome, inflammatory bowel disease, and even chronic infections or inflammation in the gut.

Additionally, people on certain medications may find themselves struggling with histamine intolerance. As mentioned, drugs like antibiotics, NSAIDs (nonsteroidal anti-inflammatory drugs), antidepressants, and muscle relaxants can inhibit DAO activity, leading to an accumulation of histamine in the body.

Histamine Intolerance: A Complex Puzzle

Understanding histamine intolerance requires piecing together a complex puzzle. It's not just about what you eat, but also about how your body processes what you eat. High-histamine foods can trigger symptoms, but so can other foods that prompt histamine release or block DAO activity. Foods like tomatoes, spinach, chocolate, and alcohol are notorious for their high histamine content. Fermented products like yogurt, sauerkraut, and soy sauce also contribute significantly to the histamine load.

Histamine intolerance is also dose-dependent. This means that small amounts of histamine might not cause any noticeable issues, but as the histamine accumulates—either through diet or the body's own production—symptoms begin to appear. This threshold varies from person to person, adding another layer of complexity to managing this condition.

Histamine intolerance is a multifaceted condition that can significantly impact your quality of life. By understanding what it is, how histamine functions in the body, the causes and mechanisms behind the intolerance, and recognizing its growing prevalence, we can take the first steps toward effective management and relief. This journey often involves meticulous tracking of symptoms, dietary adjustments, and working closely with healthcare professionals to identify and address the underlying causes.

In the chapters to come, we'll delve deeper into the symptoms of histamine intolerance, diagnostic methods, and the various strategies you can employ to manage and alleviate your symptoms. Armed with knowledge and practical tips, you'll be better equipped to navigate the challenges of histamine intolerance and reclaim control over your health and well-being.

CHAPTER 2: Symptoms of Histamine Intolerance

Histamine intolerance can manifest in a multitude of ways, affecting nearly every system in the body. Understanding these symptoms is crucial for recognizing and managing the condition effectively. In this chapter, we'll explore the common and lesser-known symptoms, offering a comprehensive view of how histamine intolerance impacts daily life.

Common Symptoms: From Headaches to Hives

One of the hallmark symptoms of histamine intolerance is headaches. These can range from mild discomfort to severe migraines that disrupt daily activities. Often, these headaches occur shortly after consuming high-histamine foods like aged cheeses, red wine, or fermented products. For some, these headaches might be accompanied by dizziness, creating a debilitating combination that can severely impact quality of life.

Skin reactions, such as hives and flushing, are another common symptom. Hives are raised, itchy welts that can appear anywhere on the body, often without an apparent trigger. Flushing, which is the sudden reddening of the skin, usually affects the face and neck. This can be particularly distressing in social situations, where the rapid onset of redness can be both visible and embarrassing.

Lesser-Known Symptoms

While headaches and skin reactions are widely recognized, histamine intolerance can present with a variety of lesser-known symptoms that often go unconnected to histamine levels. For instance, some individuals experience heart palpitations and an increased heart rate, a condition known as tachycardia. These cardiovascular symptoms can mimic those of more severe conditions, leading to unnecessary anxiety and medical testing.

Another underrecognized symptom is menstrual irregularities. Women with histamine intolerance may experience exacerbated premenstrual syndrome (PMS) symptoms, including severe cramps, bloating, and mood swings. This is due to the role histamine plays in modulating hormone levels, particularly estrogen, which can fluctuate during the menstrual cycle.

Digestive Issues: Bloating, Diarrhoea, and More

Histamine intolerance can wreak havoc on the digestive system. Bloating, a common symptom, occurs when excess gas builds up in the stomach and intestines, causing discomfort and a distended abdomen. This can be particularly troublesome after meals rich in histamine, such as smoked fish, sauerkraut, or wine.

Diarrhea is another frequent complaint. It occurs when histamine triggers excessive fluid secretion into the intestines, leading to loose, watery stools. Chronic diarrhea can result in dehydration and nutrient deficiencies if left untreated.

On the flip side, some individuals might experience constipation instead of diarrhea. This can happen due to the unpredictable nature of histamine's impact on the digestive tract, causing it to either speed up or slow down. Abdominal pain and cramping often accompany these symptoms, making mealtime a dreaded event for those affected.

Neurological Symptoms:

Anxiety, Dizziness, and Fatigue

The impact of histamine on the nervous system can lead to a variety of neurological symptoms. Anxiety is a common yet often overlooked symptom of histamine intolerance. Histamine acts as a neurotransmitter in the brain, and elevated levels can lead to feelings of anxiety, nervousness, and even panic attacks. This can create a vicious cycle, as anxiety itself can exacerbate symptoms, leading to further histamine release.

Dizziness and vertigo are also prevalent among those with histamine intolerance. These symptoms can be triggered by changes in histamine levels, affecting the inner ear and balance. The sensation of spinning or losing balance can be disorienting and frightening, particularly if it occurs frequently.

Fatigue is another debilitating symptom. This isn't the kind of tiredness that can be resolved with a good night's sleep; it's a chronic, pervasive exhaustion that affects daily functioning. Histamine intolerance can interfere with sleep quality, leading to a cycle of poor rest and increased fatigue.

Respiratory Symptoms

Congestion, Asthma, and Allergies

Histamine plays a significant role in the immune system, particularly in allergic reactions. As such, respiratory symptoms are common in those with histamine intolerance. Nasal congestion, characterized by a stuffy or runny nose, is a frequent complaint. This congestion can mimic seasonal allergies or colds, making it difficult to pinpoint histamine as the culprit.

Asthma symptoms, such as wheezing and shortness of breath, can also be exacerbated by histamine intolerance.

Histamine can cause the airways to constrict, leading to difficulty breathing. For those with pre-existing asthma, this can mean more frequent and severe attacks.

In addition to asthma and congestion, histamine intolerance can cause other allergic-type symptoms, such as sneezing, itchy eyes, and a scratchy throat. These symptoms often appear suddenly after consuming high-histamine foods or drinks, adding to the challenge of identifying the underlying cause.

Skin Reactions

Rashes, Eczema, and Flushing

Skin is often the first place where histamine intolerance manifests visibly. Rashes, which can vary from mild to severe, are common. These rashes may present as red, itchy patches that can spread across the body, causing significant discomfort.

Eczema, a chronic skin condition, can also be linked to histamine intolerance. Eczema flare-ups can result in dry, cracked skin that is prone to infection. Managing eczema often requires a combination of dietary changes and topical treatments to control histamine levels and soothe the skin.

Flushing, the sudden reddening of the skin, typically affects the face and neck. This reaction can be triggered by emotional stress, heat, or the consumption of high-histamine foods and beverages. For many, flushing is not just a cosmetic issue but a source of significant psychological distress, impacting self-esteem and social interactions.

Histamine intolerance can affect nearly every aspect of life, from physical comfort to emotional well-being. By understanding the wide range of symptoms associated with this condition, individuals can better identify and manage their histamine levels. While the journey to diagnosis and treatment can be complex, awareness is the first step towards relief and improved quality of life. Whether dealing with common symptoms like headaches and hives or navigating the challenges of lesser-known symptoms, those affected by histamine intolerance can take proactive steps to regain control over their health.

CHAPTER 3: Diagnosing Histamine Intolerance

Recognizing the Symptoms

Histamine intolerance is a chameleon-like condition, mimicking a myriad of other ailments and often leaving sufferers perplexed. Recognizing its symptoms is the first step toward effective diagnosis and treatment. The symptoms of histamine intolerance can vary widely, making it a particularly tricky condition to identify. They range from the commonplace to the obscure, encompassing almost every system in the body.

Imagine you're sitting down to a meal and within minutes, you start to feel a headache building, or perhaps your skin begins to itch inexplicably. These symptoms might seem unrelated at first glance, but they can be the hallmark of histamine intolerance. Common symptoms include headaches or migraines, digestive issues like bloating, diarrhea, and stomach cramps, as well as skin reactions such as hives, itching, or flushing. You might also experience respiratory problems like nasal congestion, asthma-like symptoms, or even heart palpitations. On a bad day, the mix of symptoms can make you feel as if you're constantly battling a flu that never fully develops.

More subtle signs include anxiety, dizziness, and fatigue. These can easily be misattributed to stress or lack of sleep, but when they occur alongside digestive disturbances or skin reactions, histamine intolerance becomes a likely suspect. Recognizing this pattern is crucial: a cluster of seemingly unrelated symptoms that flare up after eating certain foods or drinking specific beverages.

Medical History and Symptoms Assessment

Once you suspect histamine intolerance, the next step is to delve into your medical history and assess your symptoms in detail. This phase is akin to detective work, requiring meticulous documentation and analysis. Start by keeping a detailed symptom diary. Record what you eat and drink, noting the time and any subsequent symptoms. This diary becomes an invaluable tool in identifying patterns and potential triggers.

Your medical history can offer significant clues. Discuss any past experiences with allergies, food intolerances, or gastrointestinal issues with your healthcare provider. These conditions can often coexist with histamine intolerance, and a comprehensive review of your history can help to pinpoint connections. Include information about medications you are taking, as certain drugs can inhibit the enzyme diamine oxidase (DAO), which is crucial for breaking down histamine in the body.

During your assessment, consider environmental factors as well. Stress levels, exposure to allergens, and even changes in weather can influence histamine levels. By compiling all this information, you and your healthcare provider can start to see a clearer picture of how histamine intolerance affects you.

Diagnostic Tests and Procedures

Diagnosing histamine intolerance isn't straightforward, as there is no single definitive test. Instead, a combination of diagnostic approaches is often used to piece together the puzzle. Blood tests can measure histamine levels and DAO activity. Elevated histamine levels or low DAO activity can suggest histamine intolerance, but these results are not always conclusive on their own.

Another useful diagnostic tool is the skin prick test, commonly used for allergies. Although it doesn't directly diagnose histamine intolerance, it can help rule out other allergic conditions that might be causing your symptoms. The results can indicate a heightened sensitivity to histamine, providing additional evidence.

The most telling diagnostic procedure is often the elimination diet, followed by a controlled reintroduction of foods. This method, while time-consuming, offers the most direct evidence of histamine intolerance. Under the guidance of a healthcare professional, you eliminate high-histamine foods from your diet for several weeks. If your symptoms improve, histamine intolerance is likely. You then gradually reintroduce foods, one at a time, to identify which ones trigger your symptoms. Keeping a detailed food and symptom diary during this process is crucial for accurate results.

The Role of Elimination Diets in Diagnosis

The elimination diet is a cornerstone in diagnosing histamine intolerance, providing clear insights into which foods and beverages exacerbate your symptoms. It requires dedication and careful planning but can yield highly valuable information.

Begin with a list of high-histamine foods to avoid. These typically include aged cheeses, fermented products, alcohol, processed meats, and certain fish. Fresh foods are generally safer, as histamine levels increase as food ages. During the elimination phase, stick to a diet of low-histamine foods. Fresh meat, poultry, fish, eggs, certain fresh vegetables (like lettuce and zucchini), and grains like rice and quinoa are usually safe choices.

The initial phase lasts two to four weeks, allowing your body time to clear excess histamine. During this period, it's important to monitor your symptoms closely. Significant improvement often suggests histamine intolerance. Once the elimination phase is complete, you move on to the reintroduction phase. Introduce one high-histamine food at a time, eating it in moderate amounts and observing your body's reaction over the next 48 hours. This process helps to pinpoint specific triggers, offering a personalized roadmap for managing your condition.

Working with Healthcare Professionals

Navigating the complexities of histamine intolerance is best done with the support of knowledgeable healthcare professionals. Start with your primary care physician, who can refer you to specialists such as allergists, gastroenterologists, or nutritionists. Each plays a crucial role in different aspects of diagnosis and management.

Allergists can perform specific tests to rule out other allergic conditions and may offer advice on managing histamine levels. Gastroenterologists can investigate underlying digestive issues that might contribute to your symptoms, such as small intestinal bacterial overgrowth (SIBO) or leaky gut syndrome. Nutritionists or dietitians are invaluable when it comes to crafting a balanced, low-histamine diet that meets your nutritional needs without triggering symptoms.

Effective communication with your healthcare team is essential. Share your symptom diary, medical history, and any test results. Be honest about your symptoms and how they affect your daily life. This collaborative approach ensures that you receive comprehensive care tailored to your specific needs.

Diagnosing histamine intolerance is a multi-faceted process requiring a keen eye for patterns, thorough medical evaluation, and close collaboration with healthcare professionals. By recognizing the symptoms, assessing your medical history, undergoing diagnostic tests, following an elimination diet, and working with experts, you can navigate the path to effective management and improved quality of life.

CHAPTER 4: Understanding the Causes of Histamine Intolerance

Histamine intolerance can be a perplexing and frustrating condition, with symptoms that range from mildly uncomfortable to severely debilitating. To effectively manage and mitigate these symptoms, it's crucial to understand the underlying causes. In this chapter, we'll explore the complex web of factors contributing to histamine intolerance, delving into enzyme deficiencies, gut health, dietary impacts, environmental triggers, and genetic predispositions.

Enzyme Deficiencies: DAO and HNMT

Histamine intolerance often starts with a deficiency in the enzymes responsible for breaking down histamine in the body. The two primary enzymes involved are diamine oxidase (DAO) and histamine-N-methyltransferase (HNMT).

Diamine Oxidase (DAO): DAO is predominantly found in the gut and plays a critical role in breaking down dietary histamine. When DAO levels are insufficient, histamine from food can accumulate, leading to symptoms. Several factors can reduce DAO activity, including certain medications (such as antibiotics, antidepressants, and antihistamines), chronic inflammation of the gut, and gastrointestinal diseases like Crohn's disease or irritable bowel syndrome (IBS).

Histamine-N-Methyltransferase (HNMT): HNMT primarily breaks down histamine within cells, particularly in the brain, liver, and kidneys. This enzyme is crucial for metabolizing histamine released by the body in response to allergens or stress. Genetic variations can lead to reduced HNMT activity, causing an internal buildup of histamine that contributes to symptoms like headaches, fatigue, and anxiety.

Understanding enzyme deficiencies is pivotal because it highlights why some people may react severely to histamine, while others with normal enzyme levels might not.

Gut Health and Histamine Production

The gut is not just a site of nutrient absorption but also a major player in immune function and histamine regulation. Imbalances in gut health can significantly impact histamine levels in the body.

Gut Microbiota: The trillions of bacteria residing in our intestines play a crucial role in digestion and immune regulation. Dysbiosis, an imbalance in these microbial communities, can increase histamine production. Certain strains of bacteria, like Lactobacillus and Bifidobacterium, are beneficial and help regulate histamine, while others, such as Morganella morganii and

Proteus mirabilis, produce excess histamine, exacerbating symptoms.

Leaky Gut Syndrome: When the intestinal lining becomes permeable, partially digested food particles and toxins can enter the bloodstream, triggering an immune response. This condition, often referred to as "leaky gut," is associated with increased histamine production as the body attempts to defend itself against these invaders. Addressing gut permeability through diet, probiotics, and anti-inflammatory supplements can help reduce histamine levels.

The Impact of Food and Drink

Diet is a significant factor in managing histamine intolerance. Certain foods naturally contain high levels of histamine, while others can trigger histamine release in the body.

High-Histamine Foods: Foods that are aged, fermented, or processed tend to have higher histamine levels. This includes items like aged cheeses, cured meats, alcohol, and fermented products such as sauerkraut and soy sauce. Seafood, particularly if not freshly caught and consumed, can also be a major histamine source due to rapid bacterial growth and histamine production post-catch.

Histamine Liberators: Some foods don't contain much histamine themselves but can trigger the body to release its histamine stores. Examples include tomatoes, eggplants, strawberries, and certain nuts. Recognizing and limiting these foods can help manage symptoms.

Other Dietary Factors: Additives and preservatives in processed foods, artificial colors, and certain sweeteners can also contribute to histamine intolerance. Switching to a diet rich in fresh, whole foods can alleviate some of the symptoms associated with histamine intolerance.

Environmental and Lifestyle Triggers

Beyond diet, various environmental and lifestyle factors can influence histamine levels and exacerbate intolerance.

Stress: Chronic stress can increase histamine release in the body. The stress hormone cortisol can both directly and indirectly affect histamine metabolism. Finding effective stress management techniques, such as mindfulness, exercise, or hobbies, can be beneficial.

Allergens: Environmental allergens like pollen, dust mites, and pet dander can trigger histamine release as part of the immune response. Reducing exposure to these allergens through regular cleaning, air purifiers, and hypoallergenic bedding can help minimize symptoms.

Physical Activity: While moderate exercise is beneficial, intense physical activity can increase histamine release. Balancing exercise routines to avoid excessive strain can help manage histamine levels.

Temperature Changes: Extreme temperatures, whether hot or cold, can trigger histamine release in sensitive individuals. Dressing appropriately for the weather and avoiding sudden temperature shifts can help control symptoms.

Genetic Factors in Histamine Intolerance

Finally, genetics play a critical role in histamine intolerance. Variations in the genes responsible for DAO and HNMT enzyme production can affect how well these enzymes function.

Genetic Mutations: Certain genetic mutations can lead to reduced activity of the DAO or HNMT enzymes. For instance, a mutation in the AOC1 gene can result in lower DAO levels, making it difficult for the body to break down dietary histamine. Similarly, mutations in the HNMT gene can impair the breakdown of histamine within cells, leading to higher overall histamine levels.

Family History: Histamine intolerance can run in families, suggesting a genetic predisposition. If close relatives experience similar symptoms, it might indicate a hereditary component to the condition.

Epigenetics: Environmental factors and lifestyle choices can influence gene expression through epigenetic mechanisms. This means that even if you have a genetic predisposition to histamine intolerance, certain lifestyle changes and dietary adjustments can help manage symptoms by modulating gene activity.

Understanding the multifaceted causes of histamine intolerance is crucial for effective management and relief. By recognizing the roles of enzyme deficiencies, gut health, diet, environmental factors, and genetics, individuals can better tailor their approach to reducing symptoms and improving quality of life. As we continue to explore these complex interactions, ongoing research and personal experimentation will be key to finding the most effective strategies for managing histamine intolerance.

CHAPTER 5: Treatment and Management

Histamine intolerance can be a perplexing and frustrating condition to manage. The good news is that with the right strategies and knowledge, you can significantly reduce symptoms and improve your quality of life. This chapter delves into various approaches to treatment and management, focusing on dietary changes, medications and supplements, alternative therapies, and stress management.

Dietary Management: Avoiding High-Histamine Foods

One of the most effective ways to manage histamine intolerance is through careful dietary management. Histamine is found in a wide range of foods, and certain foods can trigger the release of histamine in the body.

Understanding which foods to avoid and how to structure your diet is crucial.

High-Histamine Foods to Avoid

To minimize symptoms, it's essential to avoid foods high in histamine. These include aged cheeses, fermented foods, processed meats, alcohol, and certain fish like tuna and mackerel. Leftovers can also be problematic as histamine levels increase in foods over time. Freshness is key; the fresher the food, the lower the histamine content.

Low-Histamine Alternatives

Replacing high-histamine foods with low-histamine alternatives can make a significant difference. Fresh meats and fish, most vegetables, and certain fruits like apples and pears are generally safe. Developing a meal plan that includes these safe foods ensures you maintain a balanced diet while managing your histamine levels.

Practical Tips for Dietary Management

- Plan Ahead: Meal planning can help you avoid high-histamine foods and ensure you always have low-histamine options available.

- Cook Fresh: Try to cook and eat fresh meals rather than relying on leftovers.

- Read Labels: Processed foods can often contain hidden sources of histamine. Always read labels carefully.

- Keep a Food Diary: Tracking what you eat and your symptoms can help identify specific triggers and refine your diet over time.

Medications and Supplements

While dietary management is foundational, medications and supplements can provide additional relief. These can help reduce histamine levels in the body or support the enzymes responsible for breaking down histamine.

DAO Supplements

Diamine oxidase (DAO) is an enzyme that helps break down histamine in the gut. People with histamine intolerance often have low levels of DAO. DAO supplements can be taken before meals to boost the enzyme levels and help manage symptoms. These supplements are particularly useful when eating out or consuming meals where the histamine content is uncertain.

Antihistamines

Antihistamines are commonly used to treat allergic reactions, but they can also be effective for histamine intolerance. These medications work by blocking histamine receptors, thereby reducing symptoms such as itching, hives, and nasal congestion. Non-drowsy options like loratadine and cetirizine can be taken daily, while stronger, sedating antihistamines like diphenhydramine can be used for more severe reactions.

Probiotics and Gut Health Supplements

A healthy gut is crucial for managing histamine levels. Certain probiotics can help balance gut bacteria and reduce histamine production. Probiotics like Lactobacillus rhamnosus and Bifidobacterium infantis have shown promise in managing histamine intolerance. Additionally, supplements that support gut health, such as prebiotics and digestive enzymes, can improve overall digestive function and help manage symptoms.

Alternative Therapies

Beyond conventional treatments, alternative therapies can offer additional relief and support holistic health.

Acupuncture

Acupuncture, a practice rooted in traditional Chinese medicine, involves inserting thin needles into specific points on the body. This therapy is believed to balance the body's energy flow and has been shown to reduce symptoms of histamine intolerance in some individuals. Acupuncture can help alleviate symptoms such as headaches, digestive issues, and respiratory problems.

Homeopathy

Homeopathy is a system of alternative medicine based on the principle of "like cures like." Homeopathic remedies are tailored to the individual's specific symptoms and can be effective in managing histamine intolerance. Remedies such as Histaminum, Apis mellifica, and Sulphur are often used to reduce histamine-related symptoms.

Herbal Remedies

Certain herbs have natural antihistamine properties and can help manage histamine intolerance. Quercetin, a flavonoid found in onions and apples, is a powerful natural antihistamine. Stinging nettle and butterbur are other herbs known for their anti-inflammatory and antihistamine effects. Always consult with a healthcare professional before starting any herbal remedies to ensure they are safe and appropriate for your condition.

Managing Stress and Its Impact on Symptoms

Stress can significantly impact histamine levels and exacerbate symptoms. Managing stress effectively is an integral part of treating histamine intolerance.

Mindfulness and Meditation

Practising mindfulness and meditation can reduce stress and improve overall well-being. Techniques such as deep breathing, progressive muscle relaxation, and guided imagery can help calm the mind and reduce the physical effects of stress.

Exercise

Regular physical activity is a great way to manage stress. Exercise releases endorphins, which improve mood and reduce stress. Activities like yoga, tai chi, and walking are particularly beneficial as they combine physical movement with mindfulness.

Sleep Hygiene

Adequate sleep is essential for managing stress and maintaining overall health. Establishing a regular sleep routine, creating a restful environment, and avoiding stimulants like caffeine in the evening can improve sleep quality and reduce stress.

Professional Support

Sometimes, professional support from a therapist or counsellor can be invaluable in managing stress. Cognitive-behavioural therapy (CBT) and other therapeutic approaches can provide tools and strategies to handle stress more effectively.

Managing histamine intolerance requires a multi-faceted approach that combines dietary changes, medications, alternative therapies, and stress management. By integrating these strategies into your daily routine, you can reduce symptoms and lead a healthier, more comfortable life. Remember, it's essential to work closely with healthcare professionals to tailor these treatments to your individual needs and circumstances.

CHAPTER 6: Living with Histamine Intolerance

Daily Strategies for Symptom Management

Living with histamine intolerance can seem daunting at first, but with the right strategies, you can lead a healthy, vibrant life. Managing your symptoms starts with understanding your body's unique needs and triggers. Here are some daily strategies to keep your symptoms in check.

First and foremost, maintain a food diary. Documenting what you eat and how you feel afterward can help identify which foods trigger your symptoms. Over time, you'll develop a personalised list of safe foods and those to avoid.

Hydration is another key aspect. Drinking plenty of water helps to flush out excess histamine from your system. Aim for at least eight glasses a day, and consider adding a squeeze of lemon or a splash of apple cider vinegar for a refreshing twist.

Stress management is crucial for controlling histamine levels. Practices such as yoga, meditation, and deep-breathing exercises can help keep stress in check. Exercise regularly, but avoid high-intensity workouts that might spike your histamine levels. Opt for moderate activities like walking, swimming, or cycling instead.

Ensure you get adequate sleep. Poor sleep can exacerbate histamine intolerance symptoms. Establish a regular sleep schedule and create a relaxing bedtime routine. Avoid screens an hour before bed and create a calm, dark environment to promote restful sleep.

Dietary supplements can also be beneficial. Quercetin, vitamin C, and bromelain have natural antihistamine properties and can help manage your symptoms. However, always consult with your healthcare provider before starting any new supplements.

Tips for Dining Out

Eating out can be one of the more challenging aspects of living with histamine intolerance, but with a bit of preparation, you can enjoy meals at restaurants without worry. Here are some practical tips to help you navigate dining out.

Research restaurants ahead of time. Look for places that offer customizable menus or cater to specific dietary needs. Many restaurants now provide online menus, making it easier to plan your meal choices in advance.

Don't hesitate to communicate your dietary restrictions to the restaurant staff. When making a reservation, mention your histamine intolerance and ask if the chef can accommodate your needs. Upon arrival, reiterate your dietary restrictions to your server, emphasising the importance of avoiding certain foods and ingredients.

Choose simple dishes. Opt for meals that are less likely to contain high-histamine ingredients. Grilled meats or fish with steamed vegetables, plain salads, and fresh fruit are generally safer choices. Avoid aged cheeses, cured meats, fermented foods, and dishes with heavy sauces or dressings.

If you're unsure about certain ingredients, ask your server. It's better to be safe than sorry. Most restaurants are willing to accommodate special requests, such as cooking with fresh ingredients instead of those that are pre-prepared.

Carry an emergency kit. Bring along any necessary medications or supplements you might need in case of accidental exposure to high-histamine foods. Having your essentials on hand can provide peace of mind and help manage any unexpected symptoms.

Travel Tips for Histamine Intolerance

Travelling with histamine intolerance requires some extra planning, but it shouldn't deter you from exploring the world. With these travel tips, you can enjoy your adventures while keeping your symptoms in check.

Plan ahead. Research your destination to find out about local cuisine and available dining options. Look for accommodations that offer kitchen facilities, so you can prepare your own meals if necessary. Packing non-perishable, low-histamine snacks such as rice cakes, dried fruits, and nut butters can be a lifesaver during long flights or road trips.

Pack a travel-friendly food kit. Include items like instant oatmeal packets, herbal teas, low-histamine protein bars, and portable kitchen tools like a mini blender or a travel-sized electric kettle. These can help you whip up safe, quick meals on the go.

Stay hydrated. Travelling, especially flying, can dehydrate you, which can worsen histamine intolerance symptoms. Drink plenty of water and avoid beverages like alcohol and caffeinated drinks, which can increase histamine levels.

When flying, notify the airline of your dietary needs ahead of time. Most airlines offer special meal options, and providing them with ample notice increases the likelihood of receiving a suitable meal. Pack your own meals for shorter flights to avoid any Issues.

Learn key phrases in the local language. Knowing how to communicate your dietary restrictions can be incredibly helpful, especially in countries where food allergies and intolerances are less commonly acknowledged. Phrases like "I have a histamine intolerance" or "Can this be made without [specific ingredient]?" can make dining out much easier.

Building a Support System

One of the most important aspects of managing histamine intolerance is building a robust support system. Having people who understand your condition and can offer support and advice makes a world of difference.

Start with your immediate circle. Educate your family and close friends about histamine intolerance. Explain the condition, your triggers, and what they can do to help. This not only ensures they are aware of your needs but also fosters understanding and empathy.

Join support groups, both in person and online. These groups can provide a wealth of information, from tips on managing symptoms to recommendations for healthcare providers. Sharing experiences with others who have histamine intolerance can be incredibly validating and empowering.

Seek out professional support. Work with healthcare providers who are knowledgeable about histamine intolerance. A dietitian can help you develop a safe and nutritious eating plan, while a therapist can offer strategies for coping with the emotional aspects of living with a chronic condition.

Educate yourself continuously. Stay informed about the latest research and developments in histamine intolerance. Knowledge is power, and the more you know, the better equipped you'll be to manage your condition.

Finally, don't be afraid to advocate for yourself. Whether it's at a restaurant, a social gathering, or a medical appointment, clearly communicate your needs and boundaries. Your health and well-being are paramount, and taking an active role in managing your histamine intolerance is essential.

Living with histamine intolerance may come with its challenges, but with the right strategies and support, you can lead a fulfilling and symptom-free life. Embrace these tips and make them a part of your daily routine, and you'll find yourself navigating the complexities of histamine intolerance with confidence and ease.

CHAPTER 7: Recovery and Long-Term Management

Navigating the road to recovery from histamine intolerance can feel like embarking on a challenging journey, but armed with the right knowledge and strategies, it's entirely possible to regain control of your health and well-being. In this chapter, we'll explore the timeline of recovery, the phased approach to healing, monitoring progress and adjusting strategies, long-term dietary adjustments, reintroducing foods safely, and staying informed and up-to-date with the latest developments in managing histamine intolerance.

Timeline of Recovery

Understanding the timeline of recovery is essential for managing expectations and staying motivated throughout the healing process. It's crucial to recognize that recovery from histamine intolerance is not a linear journey—progress may be gradual, with ups and downs along the way.

In the initial stages, as you begin to implement dietary changes and other treatment strategies, you may experience some relief from symptoms relatively quickly. However, full recovery often takes time and patience. It's not uncommon for individuals to see significant improvement within a few weeks to a few months of adopting a low-histamine diet and other lifestyle modifications.

For some individuals, particularly those with severe or long-standing histamine intolerance, the road to recovery may be longer and more complex. Factors such as underlying health conditions, genetic predispositions, and individual response to treatment can influence the pace and extent of recovery.

Phased Approach to Healing

Taking a phased approach to healing allows you to address histamine intolerance comprehensively and systematically. Instead of trying to implement all changes at once, breaking the process down into manageable steps can increase the likelihood of success and sustainability.

Phase one involves strict adherence to a low-histamine diet, eliminating high-histamine foods, and minimising exposure to other triggers such as alcohol, stress, and environmental allergens. During this phase, focus on identifying and removing potential sources of histamine from your diet and lifestyle.

In phase two, gradually reintroduce foods that were initially eliminated to assess tolerance levels. Keep a detailed food diary to track symptoms and reactions, and reintroduce foods one at a time, observing any changes in symptoms. Proceed cautiously, and if symptoms recur, remove the offending food and try again at a later time.

Phase three focuses on long-term maintenance and lifestyle adjustments. By this stage, you should have a good understanding of your individual triggers and how to manage them effectively. Continue to prioritize a balanced diet, stress management, adequate sleep, and regular exercise to support overall health and well-being.

Monitoring Progress and Adjusting Strategies

Monitoring your progress and adjusting strategies as needed is crucial for optimising outcomes and maintaining long-term success. Keep track of your symptoms, dietary habits, lifestyle factors, and any changes in your condition over time.

Consider keeping a symptom diary or using a mobile app to track your progress. Note any improvements or exacerbations in symptoms, as well as any deviations from your dietary or lifestyle plan. This information can help you identify patterns, triggers, and areas for improvement.

Regularly review your treatment plan with your healthcare provider or a qualified nutritionist to assess its effectiveness and make any necessary adjustments. Be open to trying new approaches or treatments based on emerging research and clinical recommendations.

Long-Term Dietary Adjustments

Making long-term dietary adjustments is essential for managing histamine intolerance effectively and preventing symptom recurrence. While strict avoidance of high-histamine foods may be necessary initially, over time, you may be able to reintroduce some of these foods in moderation.

Focus on building a diverse and nutrient-rich diet that includes a variety of fresh fruits, vegetables, lean proteins, and whole grains. Choose organic and locally sourced foods whenever possible to minimise exposure to pesticides and other contaminants.

Experiment with different cooking methods and food preparation techniques to enhance flavour and variety in your meals. Incorporate anti-inflammatory ingredients such as turmeric, ginger, and omega-3 fatty acids to support immune function and reduce inflammation.

Reintroducing Foods Safely

Reintroducing foods safely is a gradual and individualised process that requires patience and careful observation. Start by reintroducing foods that are lower in histamine and less likely to trigger symptoms, such as fresh fruits and vegetables, white rice, and certain types of meat and fish.

Monitor your symptoms closely after reintroducing each food, paying attention to any changes in digestion, energy levels, mood, and overall well-being. If symptoms occur, remove the offending food from your diet and wait until symptoms subside before trying again.

Gradually increase the complexity and diversity of foods as tolerated, but continue to avoid or limit high-histamine foods, alcohol, and other known triggers. Be prepared for some trial and error, and don't get discouraged if progress is slow or setbacks occur.

Staying Informed and Up-to-Date

Staying informed and up-to-date with the latest developments in managing histamine intolerance is essential for making informed decisions about your health. Keep abreast of current research, clinical guidelines, and expert recommendations through reputable sources such as medical journals, professional organisations, and reliable websites.

Engage with online communities, support groups, and forums to connect with others who share similar experiences and learn from their insights and strategies. Be proactive in advocating for your health and seeking out qualified healthcare providers who understand histamine intolerance and can offer personalised guidance and support.

By staying informed, proactive, and patient, you can empower yourself to take control of your health and effectively manage histamine intolerance for the long term.

In this chapter, we've explored the key principles of recovery and long-term management for histamine intolerance, including the timeline of recovery, phased approach to healing, monitoring progress and adjusting strategies, long-term dietary adjustments, reintroducing foods safely, and staying informed and up-to-date. By incorporating these strategies into your daily routine and working closely with healthcare professionals, you can optimise your chances of achieving lasting relief and reclaiming your quality of life.

CHAPTER 8: Creating a Low-Histamine Diet Plan

Embarking on a low-histamine diet journey can feel like entering uncharted culinary territory. But fear not, as we delve into the ins and outs of crafting a palate-pleasing, histamine-friendly menu that will have you savouring every bite.

Understanding Histamine Levels in Foods

Histamine levels vary widely across different foods, and having a good grasp of which foods are high, moderate, or low in histamine is essential for designing a successful low-histamine diet plan. While some foods naturally contain high levels of histamine, others may trigger histamine release in the body due to their freshness, processing, or storage methods.

Foods high in histamine include aged cheeses, cured meats, fermented foods like sauerkraut and kimchi, certain fruits such as strawberries and citrus, as well as some vegetables like tomatoes and spinach. On the other hand, low-histamine options include fresh meats, poultry, fish, most vegetables (excluding those high in histamine), gluten-free grains like rice and quinoa, dairy substitutes like almond or coconut milk, and certain fruits such as apples and pears.

Essential Low-Histamine Ingredients

Stocking your kitchen with the right ingredients is key to successfully navigating a low-histamine diet. Opt for fresh, unprocessed foods whenever possible, and steer clear of canned, fermented, or aged products. Consider incorporating these essential low-histamine ingredients into your culinary arsenal:

1. Fresh meats: Choose lean cuts of beef, poultry, and fish, and avoid processed meats like bacon or sausage.

2. Fresh fruits and vegetables: Opt for varieties that are low in histamine, such as apples, pears, broccoli, and carrots.

3. Gluten-free grains: Enjoy rice, quinoa, millet, and oats as wholesome alternatives to wheat and other gluten-containing grains.

4. Dairy substitutes: Explore the wide array of non-dairy options available, including almond milk, coconut yoghurt, and vegan cheese.

5. Fresh herbs and spices: Enhance the flavour of your dishes with fragrant herbs like parsley, basil, cilantro, and spices such as turmeric, ginger, and cinnamon.

Weekly Meal Plans for Beginners

Embarking on a low-histamine diet can feel overwhelming at first, but with careful planning and a bit of creativity, you can design a week's worth of satisfying meals that won't trigger unpleasant symptoms. Here's a sample meal plan to kickstart your journey:

Day 1:

- Breakfast: Oatmeal topped with fresh berries and a sprinkle of cinnamon

- Lunch: Grilled chicken salad with mixed greens, cucumber, and avocado

- Dinner: Baked salmon served with steamed broccoli and quinoa

Day 2:

- Breakfast: Scrambled eggs with sautéed spinach and cherry tomatoes

- Lunch: Turkey and avocado wrap with lettuce leaves instead of bread

- Dinner: Stir-fried tofu with bell peppers, snap peas, and brown rice

Day 3:

- Breakfast: Smoothie made with coconut milk, banana, and spinach

- Lunch: Quinoa salad with diced mango, cucumber, and lime vinaigrette

- Dinner: Beef stir-fry with broccoli, carrots, and snow peas served over rice noodles

Sample Meal Plan

To provide further inspiration, here's a sample meal plan for a day on a low-histamine diet:

Breakfast:

- Overnight oats made with almond milk, topped with sliced banana and a drizzle of honey

Lunch:

- Mixed green salad with grilled chicken, cherry tomatoes, cucumber, and balsamic vinaigrette

Dinner:

- Baked cod fillet seasoned with lemon and dill, served with steamed asparagus and quinoa pilaf

Delicious and Simple Low-Histamine Recipes

Preparing delicious low-histamine meals doesn't have to be complicated. Here are a few easy and flavorful recipes to add to your repertoire:

Breakfast Ideas:

- Banana and spinach smoothie: Blend together a ripe banana, a handful of spinach, almond milk, and a scoop of protein powder for a nutritious morning pick-me-up.

- Quinoa breakfast bowl: Cook quinoa according to package instructions, then top with sliced strawberries, chopped almonds, and a drizzle of maple syrup.

Lunch and Dinner Options:

- Grilled chicken Caesar salad: Toss grilled chicken breast slices with romaine lettuce, cherry tomatoes, and homemade Caesar dressing for a satisfying lunch or dinner option.

- Vegetable stir-fry: Sauté bell peppers, snap peas, and carrots in olive oil with minced garlic and ginger, then serve over brown rice for a flavorful and nutritious meal.

Snacks and Desserts:

- Apple slices with almond butter: Enjoy crisp apple slices dipped in creamy almond butter for a satisfying snack.

- Banana "nice cream": Blend frozen bananas with a splash of coconut milk until smooth, then top with chopped nuts or shredded coconut for a guilt-free dessert option.

Tips for Recipe Modifications

When adapting recipes to fit a low-histamine diet, there are a few simple modifications you can make to ensure they remain delicious and satisfying:

-Substitute high-histamine ingredients with low-histamine alternatives: Swap aged cheese for fresh mozzarella, replace tomatoes with roasted red peppers, and opt for fresh herbs instead of dried.

- Use alternative seasonings: Experiment with flavorful spices and herbs like turmeric, cumin, and basil to add depth and complexity to your dishes without relying on high-histamine ingredients.

- Focus on fresh, whole foods: Prioritise ingredients that are naturally low in histamine and avoid processed or pre-packaged foods, which may contain hidden histamines or preservatives.

By incorporating these tips and recipes into your culinary repertoire, you'll be well-equipped to design a delicious and satisfying low-histamine diet plan that supports your health and well-being. Happy cooking!

CHAPTER 9: Personal Stories and Testimonials

In the realm of health and wellness, personal experiences often carry more weight than clinical studies or medical textbooks. Real-life stories resonate deeply, providing insight, empathy, and inspiration. In this chapter, we delve into the journeys of individuals who have navigated the challenging landscape of histamine intolerance. From the initial struggles to the triumphant victories, these narratives offer a glimpse into the lives of those living with histamine intolerance.

Real-Life Experiences with Histamine Intolerance

Meet Sarah, a vibrant young woman with a zest for life. For years, Sarah battled unexplained symptoms that left her feeling fatigued, bloated, and irritable. Doctors were puzzled, running test after test without reaching a definitive conclusion. It wasn't until Sarah stumbled upon the concept of histamine intolerance that puzzle pieces began to fall into place.

"I remember the frustration of not knowing what was wrong with me," Sarah recalls. *"It was like living in a fog, never knowing when the next wave of symptoms would hit."* Through diligent research and self-experimentation, Sarah identified certain trigger foods that exacerbated her symptoms. With a newfound sense of control, she embarked on a journey of healing and discovery.

Sarah's story is not unique. Across the globe, individuals like her are sharing their experiences with histamine intolerance, forming a tight-knit community bound by empathy and understanding. Through online forums, support groups, and social media platforms, these individuals offer a beacon of hope to those still struggling to find answers.

Success Stories: Overcoming Challenges

Every journey has its challenges, but it's the triumphs that truly define us. In the realm of histamine intolerance, success stories abound, each one a testament to the power of perseverance and determination.

Take Mark, for example, a devoted father and husband who refused to let histamine intolerance dictate his life. Despite facing numerous setbacks and obstacles, Mark remained steadfast in his commitment to reclaiming his health. Through a combination of dietary modifications, stress management techniques, and targeted supplementation, Mark gradually began to experience relief from his symptoms.

"It wasn't easy," Mark admits, *"but it was worth it. Every day, I wake up feeling stronger, more energised, more alive. Histamine intolerance may have knocked me down, but it didn't keep me down."*

Mark's journey serves as a beacon of hope for countless others grappling with histamine intolerance. His story is a reminder that, with the right mindset and support system, anything is possible.

As we reflect on these personal stories and testimonials, one thing becomes abundantly clear: histamine intolerance is more than just a medical condition; it's a journey of self-discovery, resilience, and empowerment. Through the shared experiences of individuals like Sarah and Mark, we gain a deeper understanding of the challenges, triumphs, and infinite possibilities that accompany life with histamine intolerance.

We invite you to immerse yourself in the rich tapestry of human experience, to draw inspiration from those who have walked this path before you, and to embark on your own journey of healing and transformation. For in the realm of histamine intolerance, the power of the human spirit knows no bounds.

APPENDIX

In our journey through understanding histamine intolerance, it's essential to equip ourselves with the knowledge and tools necessary to navigate this condition effectively. This chapter serves as a comprehensive guide, providing clarity on essential terms, answering common questions, and offering practical resources such as food lists and a sample food diary template.

Glossary of Terms

Before delving deeper into the complexities of histamine intolerance, let's first establish a common language by exploring key terms associated with this condition. Understanding these terms will empower you to communicate effectively with healthcare professionals and fellow individuals navigating histamine intolerance.

1. Histamine: A compound produced by the body's immune system, responsible for regulating various physiological functions and triggering allergic reactions.

2. Histamine Intolerance: A condition characterised by the body's inability to properly metabolise histamine, leading to a range of symptoms when histamine levels become elevated.

3. DAO (Diamine Oxidase): An enzyme responsible for breaking down histamine in the body, commonly deficient in individuals with histamine intolerance.

4. HNMT (Histamine N-Methyltransferase): Another enzyme involved in histamine metabolism, deficiencies of which can contribute to histamine intolerance.

5. Mast Cells: Cells of the immune system that release histamine and other inflammatory compounds in response to allergens and other triggers.

6. *Allergen*: A substance that triggers an allergic reaction in sensitive individuals, potentially leading to the release of histamine.

7. *Elimination Diet:* A dietary approach aimed at identifying and removing potential triggers, such as high-histamine foods, to alleviate symptoms and pinpoint intolerances.

8. *Symptom Threshold:* The level of histamine exposure at which symptoms of histamine intolerance become noticeable or problematic for an individual.

9. *Histamine Receptor Antagonist:* Medications that block histamine receptors, commonly used to alleviate symptoms of allergies and histamine intolerance.

10. Probiotics: Beneficial bacteria that support gut health and may play a role in histamine metabolism and immune function.

11. Histamine Sensitivity: Another term used interchangeably with histamine intolerance, referring to the body's heightened reactivity to histamine due to impaired metabolism or excessive histamine levels.

12. Histamine Liberators: Substances that stimulate the release of histamine from mast cells, potentially exacerbating symptoms of histamine intolerance. Examples include alcohol, certain medications, and some food additives.

13. Histamine Blockers: Another term for histamine receptor antagonists, medications that block the action of histamine at its receptors, thereby reducing symptoms of allergies and histamine intolerance.

14. DAO Inhibitors: Substances that inhibit the activity of diamine oxidase (DAO), the enzyme responsible for breaking down histamine in the gut. DAO inhibitors can contribute to elevated histamine levels and worsen symptoms of histamine intolerance.

15. Histidine: An amino acid found in protein-rich foods that serves as a precursor to histamine. Histidine levels in foods can influence histamine levels in the body, making it relevant to histamine intolerance.

16. Mast Cell Activation Syndrome (MCAS): A condition characterised by abnormal mast cell activation and release of histamine and other inflammatory compounds, leading to symptoms similar to histamine intolerance.

17. Histamine Clearance: The process by which histamine is metabolised and eliminated from the body, primarily through the actions of DAO and HNMT enzymes.

18. Histamine Receptors: Proteins located on the surface of cells that bind to histamine, initiating cellular responses that contribute to allergic reactions and inflammation. There are four main types of histamine receptors, each with distinct functions and distribution in the body.

19. Histamine Containing Foods: Foods that naturally contain histamine or histamine-releasing compounds, contributing to histamine levels in the body and potentially triggering symptoms in individuals with histamine intolerance.

20. Histamine Degradation Pathway: The biochemical pathway involved in the breakdown and elimination of histamine from the body, encompassing enzymatic reactions mediated by DAO, HNMT, and other factors.

By familiarising yourself with these terms, you'll be better equipped to navigate discussions, research, and treatment options related to histamine intolerance.

Frequently Asked Questions

When confronted with a complex health condition like histamine intolerance, it's natural to have questions. Here, we address some of the most common inquiries to provide clarity and peace of mind.

1. What are the typical symptoms of histamine intolerance?

- Common symptoms include headaches, digestive issues (such as bloating and diarrhoea), neurological symptoms (such as anxiety and fatigue), respiratory symptoms (such as congestion and asthma), and skin reactions (such as rashes and flushing).

2. How is histamine intolerance diagnosed?

- Diagnosis often involves a combination of recognizing symptoms, medical history assessment, symptom tracking, and possibly diagnostic tests such as serum DAO levels or elimination diets.

3. What foods should I avoid if I have histamine intolerance?

- High-histamine foods such as aged cheeses, fermented foods, processed meats, and certain fruits and vegetables are commonly avoided. Additionally, foods that stimulate histamine release or inhibit DAO production should be minimised.

4. Are there any medications or supplements that can help manage histamine intolerance?

- Yes, DAO supplements, antihistamines, and probiotics are commonly used to support histamine metabolism and alleviate symptoms.

5. Can histamine intolerance be cured?

- While histamine intolerance cannot be cured, symptoms can often be effectively managed through dietary adjustments, lifestyle changes, and targeted supplementation.

6. Is histamine intolerance the same as a food allergy?

- No, histamine intolerance is distinct from a food allergy. While both involve adverse reactions to certain foods, histamine intolerance is characterised by the body's inability to properly metabolise histamine, whereas food allergies involve an immune response to specific allergens.

By addressing these frequently asked questions, we aim to provide clarity and empower individuals to take control of their health and well-being despite the challenges of histamine intolerance.

Comprehensive Food Lists: High and Low Histamine Foods

One of the cornerstones of managing histamine intolerance is understanding which foods to include and which to avoid. Below, we provide comprehensive lists of high and low histamine foods to guide your dietary choices.

High Histamine Foods:

- Aged cheeses (such as blue cheese, cheddar, and parmesan)

- Fermented foods (such as sauerkraut, kimchi, and kombucha)

- Processed meats (such as bacon, salami, and hot dogs)

- Smoked and cured meats (such as smoked salmon and ham)

- Shellfish (such as shrimp, crab, and lobster)

- Certain fruits (such as strawberries, bananas, and citrus fruits)

- Certain vegetables (such as tomatoes, spinach, and eggplant)

- Alcohol (especially red wine and beer)

- Vinegar and vinegar-containing foods (such as pickles and mustard)

- Certain condiments and sauces (such as soy sauce and ketchup)

Low Histamine Foods:

- Fresh meats (such as chicken, turkey, and fresh fish)

- Fresh fruits (such as apples, pears, and berries)

- Fresh vegetables (such as broccoli, carrots, and leafy greens)

- Gluten-free grains (such as rice, quinoa, and oats)

- Dairy alternatives (such as almond milk and coconut yoghourt)

- Non-fermented soy products (such as tofu and edamame)

- Herbs and spices (such as parsley, basil, and turmeric)

- Cooking oils (such as olive oil and coconut oil)

- Certain grains (such as rice and millet)

- Sweeteners (such as honey and maple syrup)

By referencing these lists, individuals with histamine intolerance can make informed choices when planning meals and grocery shopping, helping to minimise symptom triggers and promote overall well-being.

Sample Food Diary Template

Keeping a food diary can be a valuable tool for identifying patterns and pinpointing potential triggers of histamine intolerance. Below is a sample food diary template to help you track your dietary intake and associated symptoms:

Date:

Meal/Food Item:
- Description of the meal or food item consumed

Quantity/Serving Size:
- Amount consumed (e.g., number of servings, portion size)

Time:
- Time of consumption (e.g., breakfast, lunch, dinner, snack)

Symptoms Experienced:
- List any symptoms experienced after consuming the meal or food item (e.g., headache, bloating, skin rash)

Notes:
- Additional comments or observations related to the meal or food item (e.g., preparation method, specific ingredients)

By consistently recording your dietary intake and associated symptoms using this template, you can gain valuable insights into your body's response to different foods and beverages, facilitating targeted dietary adjustments and symptom management.

In conclusion, this chapter serves as a comprehensive guide for navigating histamine intolerance, offering clarity on essential terms, answering common questions, and providing practical resources to support individuals in managing their condition effectively. Armed with knowledge and tools, you can embark on your journey toward improved health and well-being despite the challenges posed by histamine intolerance.

* 9 7 9 8 3 2 6 8 0 4 2 1 1 *